SPIR & DUS

Death is a Dialogue between
The Spirit and the Dust.
"Dissolve," says Death — The Spirit, "Sir,
I have another Trust" —

Emily Dickinson

SPIRIT
&
DUST

MEDITATIONS
for WOMEN with DEPRESSION

Maura Hanrahan

SPIRIT & DUST
Meditations for Women with Depression
by Maura Hanrahan

Note: In the course of my depression I availed of support services in two countries. I have met many women (and men) who were depressed, and I have read
a lot about other people's experience of depression. 1 have also participated
in a twelve-step program as well as support groups for women suffering from
depression. Some of the vignettes that follow in this book come from the experiences of other women with their depression. In all cases — except my own
— names and other details have been changed to protect the identities of the
women. My focus is on the meaning of these stories and experiences, not their
specific circumstances, and this is what I have tried to convey.

Edited by Gregory F. Augustine Pierce
Cover by Tom A. Wright
Cover art, "Woman," by Maura Hanrahan
Text design and typesetting by Patricia A. Lynch

Published by ACTA Publications, 5559 W. Howard Street,
Skokie, IL 60077-2621, (800) 397-2282, www.actapublications.com

Library of Congress Catalog number: 2009925185
ISBN: 978-0-87946-396-0
Printed in the United States of America by Versa Press
Year 20 19 18 17 1615 14 13 12 11 10 09
Printing 15 14 13 12 11 10 9 8 7 6 5 4 3 2 First

♲ Text printed on 30% post-consumer recycled paper

CONTENTS

DEDICATION

For Paul and Jemma

PROLOGUE

"De-pres-sion." Three innocent syllables make up such a benign-sounding word. It conjures up images of a downward slope in a road or a slump in the stock market. It suggests something passing, even fleeting: certainly a temporary thing to get through on the way to somewhere else. It's hardly evocative of the cancerous nature of the condition, a still-mysterious illness that can wound, damage, and even kill. Depression snakes through once-solid marriages, injects poison into workplaces and careers, and rips lives to pieces.

In the 1930s, they recognized the inadequacy of the word and had the good sense to put "Great" before it. They knew "depression" was just too mild, too insufficient, for a phenomenon that engulfed people. Maybe what we are going through right now is the "Almost-Great" Depression (or maybe it will turn into the "Greater Than the Great" Depression).

More than a groove in an otherwise smooth road, depression is a giant pothole in the making. At first, it might be a dip in a green valley or a sour mood that refuses to be shaken off.

It can become a maelstrom that grips us entirely. It alternates between a blizzard of despair and the aridness of a desert, not a Joshua tree in sight. In either case, the ground is rarely level and it feels like it might be swept away at any moment. Put bluntly, depression is hellish and can kill you.

Depression — "mind storm" might be a more apt phrase — is among the worst things that can happen to you. Later, when its waters have long receded, it seems that it might also be one of the best.

I suffer from depression. I have also learned from it. I could not have written this little book otherwise. But this book is about you, not about me, and so I have described my own journey with the disease for those who might want to read it. It is in the Epilogue at the end of the book.

What I want you to read are these meditations, as often and in whatever order you please, in the hope that they will help you deal with the "spirit and dust" of depression.

The wisdom of Christian women mystics has been a real palliative for me in dealing with my depression. These are women from the tenth century right up to our own. Among them are Blessed Julian of Norwich, who lived much of her life cloistered in a "cell" in England; Julian's friend, Margery Kempe; Saint Jane de Chantal, a wise, motherly religious leader from France; American poet Anne Bradshaw; and the lively Edwina Gateley, who works with women on the margins today.

Many of these women lived with illness, including depression. On a daily basis, they were part of societies and a church that saw them as second class — not as good as men, the descendants of Adam's rib and Eve's sin, if you like. At times they lost sight of God and felt deserted by God. Other times they were almost over-powered by the love of God. Their problems were ours; their lives were ours. In their words there is much wisdom, love, and healing. Spending time with them has helped me close some of my wounds, slowly but surely. Sit with the women mystics awhile. There, I hope you will find some solace and respite.

Father, pour the oil of Your bountiful mercy on my wounds, for You are my only hope; heal me.

Saint Jane de Chantal

IGNORANCE

Why, if there is so much information available, do we not know about depression? Is it a secret? A conspiracy of silence? Or is it just that no one cares? Or that we are afraid to talk about it?

One in eight people will be hospitalized for depression during their lifetime. One in ten adults will experience depression. In the United States alone, this is no less than nineteen million people. Some of them will die from this illness.

After eight years of university education, including graduate school, however, I knew virtually nothing about depression, even though most of these years had been spent in the study of the social sciences. I attended three universities — three thriving, lively educational facilities in two different countries. I walked across three different stages to collect diplomas representing three degrees. I was hyper-educated, yet my ignorance of this reality for so many people, especially women, was practically boundless.

What a shock when I became depressed myself. I had no clue what was even happening to me, much less what do to about it. As I finally came to grips with my diagnosis, I discovered that depression is a complete mystery to almost everyone I know.

My cell will not be one of stone or wood
but of self-knowledge.

Saint Catherine of Siena

PMS

"PMS. That's your problem," the chubby, jocular doctor says, chuckling. "It'll pass."

He brushes his thinning hair back over the top of his head. He tucks his stethoscope in the pocket of his white coat and ushers me to the door that leads back out to his waiting room. "Back to the cold, cold world," a voice says in my head.

Never mind that this PMS episode goes on from January 1st until New Year's Eve, never taking a vacation or even an afternoon off.

Surely a woman doctor will understand and make better sense of it: This one has blue eyes and I search them for any sign of kindliness, but it isn't there.

"It's part of a woman's life," the woman doctor says. "You just have to get used to it."

My eyes can hardly focus as I walk down the stairs from her office. In the dismissiveness of her words, I hear judgment, an insinuation of inadequacy, and an impatience with my impatience.

What if she is right? Then what? This is normal? This is how a woman's life is lived?

My blood, my woman's blood, freezes in my veins.

From now on, I put myself in your divine hands.
Do what you like with me.

Saint Teresa of Los Andes

MISSING GOD

Where is God? Not in the pink and yellow roses in the little shop on the corner, not in a husband's deep kiss or in the downy fur of a small kitten.

Where is God? God can no longer be found in a stream of words on paper or in lush paint on canvas. God is not in the bread that sits on our tongues, the water that flows down our throats, or the air that puffs up our lungs. There is a deadness to all these things, these things that give life.

Without God, there is no almighty protector, no giver of life and of comfort. There is only aloneness. There is no mother, no father, no sister, no brother, no partner with warm arms that embrace and hold. Without God, there is no solace even in the silence and stillness; there is just an empty barren ground stretching on for miles, the echoes hollow.

If God is gone, there is nothing. One who cannot feel the presence of God is as naked and helpless as a newborn mouse. And, unlike the baby mouse, one has a keen awareness that this is so.

Who is this maker, lover and sustainer God? I do not have the words to express it. Until I am united with God, I can never have true rest or peace. I can never know until I am held so close to God that there is nothing between us.

Blessed Julian of Norwich

HELPLESSNESS

Slowly swirls of steam rise up from the pot. They're white and ghost-like, little tendrils that dissipate as they reach higher. The water that has birthed them rumbles, growls, and finally boils. Soon it's at fever pitch.

The water moans and pasta bobs in the water. Once hard and curly, it now slackens by the second. As the noise increases, the ribbons of stream rise further. Then there is a volcano of bubbles.

Dinner is done.

But my body has become catatonic, as immoveable as cast concrete. The bubbles seem to shout now. Finally they begin to climb out of the pot, sloshing over the stovetop, hissing along the way.

Still, I can do nothing but watch. Something has taken hold of my spirit and the weakened body that houses it. There is too only numbness and no opening for fear.

God said not, "You shall not be tempested, you shall not be afflicted," but "You shall not be overcome."

Blessed Julian of Norwich

TEMPTING FATE

My habit of crossing the street slowly in London was a kind of flirtation with golden-crowned, scythe-carrying Santa Muerte. The city bulged with people, every single one of whom seemed to be in a mad tear to get to some unknown destination. They jumped in and out of fumes-spewing cars and buses as if they were being chased. In the crazy morning hours, vehicles created an intimidating blur on the Commercial Road and the Strand.

This habit was not a planned thing, it was unexpected, like a ghoul that suddenly popped out of the shadows and overpowered me. Walk when the light flashes "don't walk." Wave away the cab driver who screeches, "Are you retarded?" Hope it ends, hope it doesn't, hope to at least wake up in a hospital with kindly nurses and concerned doctors.

It was not unreasonable to expect an "accident" there, given that the British drive on the left side of the road, jarring North American residents of their country, of which I was a temporary one.

But there was a surprise in all this, too. Despite their dizzying speeds, most of the drivers were more careful than I expected. It was always frustratingly easy to reach the other side of the street safely.

Death is a Dialogue between
The Spirit and the Dust.
"Dissolve," says Death — The Spirit, "Sir,
I have another Trust" —

Emily Dickinson

FEAR
of the
MARKETPLACE

It turns out that this other thing, my other persistent eccentricity, has got a name as well: agoraphobia. It's from the Greek and literally means "fear of the marketplace"; it really means fear of any place that people gather — which is just about everywhere outside my little living room.

"Fear of the marketplace," the dictionary calmly explains. It's virtually impossible to keep from laughing because, oddly enough, the marketplace is one of the few places that still feels relatively safe and welcoming to me. It is even an enjoyable place to be at times, like a vestige of a life that seems so long ago and even elusive now.

The vendors have sing-song voices — "Fresh bananas! Juicy apples, MacIntosh, Pippens! Get 'em here!" These voices carry a comfort in them, like the soft blankets we lugged around as toddlers. There is soothing, too, in the verdancy of the bell peppers and the sunshine yellow of the bananas. The eye can focus on these things, allowing the mind to block out the screaming horrors that sometimes seem all around.

Agoraphobia is "common" among women, according to the cold paragraphs in an otherwise upbeat magazine. It's associated with panic attacks: fluttering tummies; quick, rasping, shallow breath; and hands that have their own internal earthquake. The only relief is to stay inside, away from anything that might trigger this particular tsunami. And that is just what we sufferers do. In some cases, the article informs us, homes become prisons for years on end. It is not encouraging.

But giving something a name feels like a step forward, a tiny one, but a step forward nevertheless. It's like water, though: hard to hold onto.

Then again, labels can make you mercilessly cruel to yourself. Already depressed, you start to think of yourself as defective, weak, in the bleakest moments, a freak. The magazine offers no advice, no solutions, and very little hope. Staying indoors most of the time isn't so bad anyway.

May the angel of God precede you, and the son of God protect you, and his mother guard you.

Blessed Hildegard of Bingen

HELPMATES

In the fairy tales, the prince rescues the imprisoned princess from the tower. She's a bit helpless, or she's been made that way, and he is a problem-solver. He knows just what to do to make things better.

When a princess needs rescuing (of whatever kind), many men want to make like the prince. They know, deep down, that this is what is expected of them.

Well, this damsel in distress would love to be rescued. Her husband would love to rescue her. He is desperate to make everything all right. He beats himself up because his consistent, monumental efforts to help don't amount to much.

He feels like he is failing the woman who loves and needs him. He's so frustrated that he runs around like a chicken with his head cut off. Sometimes he snaps at small questions or interrupts when it is least wanted. (No more than the damsel in distress does, mind you.)

The husband is almost as trapped in her depression as his wife is. He is certainly as confounded by it as she is. He knows that sufferer Winston Churchill called it "the black dog"; he's immersed himself in the pages of William Styron's *Darkness Visible*. He understands how persistent this ghastly condition is and he is afraid, too. Sometimes he wants to scream 'til his lungs are empty.

He wants our family life back.

"Write about how husbands want to fix things," he says. "Explain how bad we feel when we can't."

Love transforms you into what you love.

Saint Catherine of Siena

TEARS

The night was spent in tears. Lacking boxed tissues, I relied on a roll of toilet tissue, and now all that is left is the cardboard cylinder. I could not stop crying. No one died; I didn't fail an exam or lose a job; I didn't battle with my husband or fall out with a girlfriend. There is no identifiable reason for these tears, but they had a mind of their own.

Today my eyes are so swollen I can barely open them. I peer through the slits at the mirror. Hopelessness washes over me, followed by embarrassment and shame. My cheeks are puffed up like mushroom clouds, sore from the steady stream of salt that assaulted them through the dark hours.

Something is banging the inside of my skull; it's as if I drank half a bottle of vodka the night before (though I didn't). There is nothing I can do today — going out in public looking like this is not an option. And I'm not capable of getting myself dressed and out the door anyway.

I know this will be one of the horrible days. I won't be able read or watch TV with my eyes like this. The radio is the only possible way to pass time.

I am desperate for something to do. Otherwise I'll beat myself up all day for such irrational behavior and for the costly consequences of it. There was no gain from those tears, no compensation — just pure, bleak waste.

From now on, I put myself in your divine hands.
Do what you like with me.

Saint Teresa of Los Andes

TERROR

The morning alarm clock brings the kind of terror you might feel as a Mack truck hurtles toward you, with your feet inexplicably glued to the concrete. Fright hormones rush through my veins, up and down my body, from the top of my head to my little toe. The terror creates a thunder in my heart. Instead of smooth breaths in and out, there is only a thin whistle of air.

My husband's warm presence, only a few inches away, means absolutely nothing. His loving gaze does not register; it is as if he is speaking a foreign language I have never heard. Only intellect can remind me that he is my family, my beloved of all beloveds.

But right now I sure don't want to talk to him. I wish he'd go away and leave me alone. I am busy summoning up my remaining shreds of strength necessary to deal with the onrushing terror.

The mantras start: Try to concentrate; remember you're not alone; know that everything will be all right, that there's really nothing to be afraid of.

Repeat mantras. Repeat mantras. Repeat mantras.

Slowly the terror falls away, like a meteor from the sky.

For just a nano-second there is the strongest sense that I could not have done it alone.

I am your child, all yours.

Saint Jane de Chantal

NEEDINESS

Oh to be a soft-skinned baby, new to the world, unknowing, unaware of any darknesses that might become visible later. Sinking into blissful sleep, untroubled, unworried, unthinking. Then moving gently into wakefulness and calling for warm nourishment, anticipating the wet comfort of it in my throat.

Feeling strong arms underneath my body, rocking back and forth, like the branches of willow trees in a gentle summer breeze.

Gurgling, chuckling, smiling, laughing. As if there is nothing else to do in the world.

Happiness. Pure happiness. Only happiness.

Mother, my mother.

Saint Paula Montal

NO REASON

There are diplomas on my wall, proudly tucked into firm black frames. The refrigerator is stuffed with carrots, potatoes, zucchini, apples, skinless chicken breast, fresh sole. There are condiments of every sort, even tongue-tickling chili sauce. Outside, a reliable car sits in the driveway, always ready to take me for a leisurely spin or a trip to the drugstore or supermarket. To my husband's great relief, the roof in this house doesn't leak.

True, the walls are dull beige, but less than a mile away there is all manner of paint and wallpaper available should we choose to change them. There is money in the bank. Not tons, but enough. In this country, medical care remains free and accessible, despite media hysteria to the contrary just south of the border.

Most people would look at this picture and see something close to perfection. So there is no obvious reason for my despair and the paralysis that accompanies it. There is no apparent need for the floods of tears that mark my every single day. There is really nothing to worry about.

My affliction, if that's what it is, makes no obvious sense. I should count my blessings. That's the message I receive. According to every television commercial and the more subtle messages that surround me at every turn, someone in my position has it "all" and, therefore, should be happy.

Mystery of mysteries: A woman can sit in her safe, pretty living room and feel the thirst of being lost in the desert.

With regard to mental preoccupations: Without worrying about them, try to remain calm amid this warfare of distractions. Just sit there, convinced that this patience is a powerful prayer before God.

Saint Jane de Chantal

GUILT

Some of us feel we have no right to be depressed. But there is no denying the fact of the depression itself and its stubborn persistence.

Guilt washes over me like lava pouring out of a volcano. Octopus-like, it wraps me in its long, cold, slimy tentacles; its grip is firm.

Depression has no mercy. The guilt it induces is a steel trap, catching its victims triumphantly, squeezing hope and life out of us.

The guilt fills all available space and pushes away any vestiges of peace, any glimpse of serenity. "You have no right to feel this way," it screams, its voice never deteriorating to hoarseness and quiet.

Guilt throws up images of malnourished children with swollen bellies, single mothers struggling the pay the rent, bent-over men queuing up at city shelters. Our parents and teachers were fond of repeating the old proverb that there is always someone worse off, and now it is as if this proverb is in the room, its arms crossed in front of its chest.

Guilt steps between us and our suffering. It is sharp-edged and dangerous. It is as frightening as it is oppressive.

For I saw no wrath except on man's side,
and He forgives that in us.

Blessed Julian of Norwich

SHAME

Guilt is always accompanied by shame. And shame is as corrosive to the soul as rust is to metal.

Shame is like a tornado, over-powering everything in its path, wrecking all it touches. Shame is a mix of loathing and hatred, but this concoction is not directed outward; it is reserved for ourselves. Shame is even crueler than guilt and has less even mercy. Shame, it quickly becomes clear to anyone suffering from depression, has the ultimate power, the power to kill.

Our usual inner resources are not functional or available when we are depressed. Depression means that the reptile in the brain is in charge, running amok with heartless abandon. It's hard to sir the intellect to wakefulness, much less to action.

But eventually adrenalin helps. In its largely unrecognized brilliance, the body usually offers us some sort of life raft. A rush of adrenalin often leads not to panic; instead, it kick-starts the mind. "Don't give in to Shame," whispers a distant voice. "Pretend you are fine. Fake it."

It's not a perfect solution, but it might keep the Shame from committing the murder it is crying out to commit.

Do not worry about your perfection, or about your soul. God, to whom it belongs, and to whom you have completely entrusted it, will take care of it and fill it with all the graces, consolation and blessings of His holy love.

Saint Jane de Chantal

DIAGNOSIS

Finally, after a raft of visits to doctors, my condition has a name. Or, more properly, a diagnosis. It's not me. There is nothing wrong with *me*. It's an illness. It's a medical phenomenon, meaning it's something that happens to other people, too. I'm not alone in this; there are others out there somewhere.

"I'm pretty sure you're depressed," the doctor says simply and straightforwardly. He's a psychiatrist. He must know. He does, he assures me. He's seen hundreds of people like me.

The doctor has kind brown eyes and silver-streaked hair that lends him even more credibility. "I'd call it major depression," he adds. It's hard not to notice the calm in his voice. He's almost casual, but it's reassuring rather than disrespectful.

I've said nothing — I'm still trying to drink in the knowledge that I am ill — but he continues: "The good news is there are things we can do about it."

He stops and looks right into my eyes, probably to make sure I'm listening. "I'm going to write out a prescription that is very effective for most people," he says.

I nod. Then he explains that it will take up to six weeks for the medication to take effect. It's tempting to spit out a cynical remark, something about punishing the depressed, but I take a pass. This is the best news I've had in a long time, and it's more useful to focus on it.

As I walk down the corridor, leaving his office behind, a strange feeling washes over me. It's kind of foreign, or like a friend you haven't seen for a long, long time. It's Relief, and it's almost enough to make me smile.

Now I shall drink wisdom from the spruces'
*   sap-filled crowns,*
now I shall drink truth from the withered
*   trunks of the birches,*
now I shall drink power from the smallest
*   and tenderest grasses:*
a mighty protector mercifully reaches me his hand.

Edith Södergran

RELIEF

There is almost a skip in my step when I think of my diagnosis of depression. Isn't that "crazy"? But perhaps I have found Sweet Relief at last. There's an almost imperceptible increase in my energy; it's minute, but it's there and so very welcome.

It's been only twenty-four hours since I was diagnosed, and it's almost as if my depression has been cured. But, of course, this is not the case. It's not long before the sharp edge of psychological pain cuts into my psyche once again. The mind storm begins, and an all-out crying jag takes hold of me and shakes me from my spine.

Then disillusionment and hopelessness set in. The latter feeling is familiar, and now it swamps me. The diagnosis represented a light at the end of a long, damp, closed-in tunnel, but now it is barely flickering.

Is everything slipping away?

That night sleep comes at my bidding, however. That in itself is an unusual gift my body and soul have been crying out for. In the morning, there is a flash of insight: The diagnosis is only step one; I am a baby who has just taken her first tentative step.

All shall be well, and all shall be well
and all manner of things shall be well.

Blessed Julian of Norwich

SHOCK

My father is astonished. No one in his family ever saw a psychiatrist before, he says. What about my cousins, Barbara, Andrea....? I list two or three more. He's visited them in the psychiatric ward, for goodness' sake. And what about my aunt June?

But he means *his* family: his wife and his children, the nuclear family that he is responsible for making happy. This can't be happening; it wasn't part of his plan; it means he might have failed one of his children.

The local mental health association has a pamphlet for family members. As he reads it, his eyes widen. Depression is amazingly common, he learns. It is, in fact, all around us, although we usually fail to see it.

A traditional man in many ways, Dad looks at me as if he has never seen me before. He doesn't understand what is happening to me. But, then, neither do I.

But I and those who loved me wondered why
such great persecution came upon me, and why
God did not bring me comfort.

Blessed Hildegard of Bingen

LEARNING

Now begins a learning process. It turns out that there is abundant material on depression at the library. An entire shelf in the city's biggest bookstore is dedicated to the disease. It's hard not to be overwhelmed by all the books and magazine and journal articles. It's difficult to know where to start.

"Somewhere" is the answer. "Anywhere" is another. So is "here": a simple pamphlet from the National Institute of Mental Health, part of the United States' National Institutes of Health network.

There are three types of depression, it says. "Bipolar condition," once known as "manic-depression," is the least common. Sufferers of this type of depression alternate between disturbing highs and lows. Their lives can be a jarring cycle of euphoria, hyperactivity, and irresponsibility coupled with sadness, despair, and even suicidal thoughts and behaviors. Men and women have the same rate of bipolar illness, but women tend to have more of the depressive symptoms.

The condition is a cruel one, and many women have made huge financial, relationship, and sexual mistakes during their "high" or out-of-control phases. One woman I know drained her bank account and bought a shiny red Camaro with cash. Another slept with an office mate she normally disliked. A third crashed her car at a shocking speed in the middle of the night. She hadn't slept in days. Now she has spinal injuries to deal with.

"Dysthymia" is a milder form of depression that lasts at least two years. People with dysthymia are joyless and often tired. This is often considered to be "just their personalities." They can, however, develop major depression.

Major depression is probably the most common and well known of the depressive illnesses. (This is not to say it's understood, accepted, or easily diagnosed or treated.) It lasts from a few weeks to many years, especially if it is not diagnosed early. Most major depressions last several months or longer. According to the National Institute of Mental Health, depression is "a pervasive and impairing illness."

So, courage, my dear ones.

Saint Jane de Chantal

SYMPTOMS
of
MAJOR DEPRESSION

The symptoms of major depression:

- A persistent sad, anxious or "empty" mood.
- Loss of interest in activities, including sex.
- Irritability and excessive crying.
- Sleeping too much or too little, with early morning wakening.
- Guilt, hopelessness, and worthlessness.
- Loss of appetite or weight loss or overeating and weight gain.
- Fatigue and a feeling of being "slowed down."
- Difficulty concentrating, remembering, and making decisions.
- Physical symptoms that persist and don't respond to treatment.
- Suicidal thoughts or actions.

There's a liberating recognition in this list, but also an enveloping feeling of isolation and fear. How not to drown in information?

I give you my eyes that you may see all things with them, and my ears, that you may hear all things with them; my mouth I also give you, so that all you have to say, whether in speech, prayer, or song, you may say through it. I give you my heart, that through it you may think everything and may love me and all things for my sake.

Saint Mechtilde von Hackeborn

WOMEN'S BODIES

In the locker room after swimming, the women joke about women's woes. We all do this: women who came with their best friends, others who come alone but easily join in.

"God must be a man because he gave women periods," Sophie laughs, telling an old, old joke.

The cards do seemed stacked against us, we all sigh.

"Men have it easy," says Lynn. We all nod at this fundamental truth (it is a fundamental truth for us, anyway).

Our bantering is a form of female bonding. It's also a way of dealing with the odd truth that we are the ones who have to cope with menstrual periods, pregnancy, childbirth, and then menopause. Life seems so steady for men; their bodies seem so reliable.

Women experience depression at a rate that is twice as high as men's. This rate exists regardless of race, ethnic background, or socioeconomic status. This is true all over the world.

Why?

Daughters of Israel, God raised you from beneath
The tree, so now remember how it was planted.
Therefore rejoice, daughters of Jerusalem!

Blessed Hildegard of Bingen

CYNICISM

Depression is "a highly treatable illness," reads the brochure. It isn't hard to picture a satisfied, chirpy woman clicking these words onto her keyboard. "I'm too blessed to be depressed," she might have written. Her half-glasses sit on her nose as she peers over them to double-check what she's written. Her peers will review this, comment on it, critique it, and validate it. They'll sign off, and it will go to the printers. From coast to coast across the continent, depressed people will read it. And get more depressed.

Then what? Clearly, this woman and her colleagues have never been through my hell. They don't know what they're talking about.

Ah, my full-on cynicism has returned.

"Treatment is effective for over 80% of cases." Sure, it is. Yet the same brochure even admits that no two people experience depression in exactly the same way. So there!

Maybe there is an anti-depression industry out there, a Military-Industrial Complex for the Depressed, creating high-paying jobs for this woman and others like her.

But the rest of the woman's words beckon. "Realize that your negative feelings are part of depression," she writes. "And don't expect too much from yourself right away."

Maybe that lady in front of the computer screen really is thinking of us as she types. Maybe she does know what she is talking about. Maybe she does care.

Anyone who has waded
Through love's turbulent water,
Now feeling hunger and now satiety,
Is untouched by the season
Of withering or blooming,
For in the deepest
And most dangerous waters,
On the highest peaks,
Love is always the same.

Hadewijch of Antwerp

(translated by Oliver Davies)

WHY?

Over and over, one short simple word pops up in the minds of us depressed women. It is a word that proliferates like dandelions in spring: "Why?" We know that bad things happen to good people, but we don't know why this, of all things, has happened to us, of all people.

Teams of dedicated people in white coats attempt to answer this question, and their theories can become a refuge for those of us who suffer.

Biological vulnerability to depression may be inherited, they say. But they suspect other factors are involved as well. Biochemistry is important; neurotransmitters or certain brain chemicals aren't working properly.

Increasingly, there is attention being paid to environmental factors: the death of a partner or friend; the loss of a cherished job; physical illness, like the common disease of hypothyroidism; or maybe something as traumatic as having one's house burglarized. All these can trigger, if not cause, depression.

About one-third of people with depression have substance-abuse problems, but this "why" begs the proverbial question: Which came first, the chicken or the egg? Did the depressed person take up drinking or gambling as a way of coping with the depression? Or did the bottle or the casino or both lead to the depression.

A similar question has to be asked when the literature cites low self-esteem and pessimistic thinking as factors in depression. Am I depressed because I think poorly of myself and my propects, or is it the other way around?

Some of the research and analysis is nothing more than common sense. But the truth about our own depression is always a quagmire with no satisfactory answer in sight.

I belong to God. He created me
and is my beginning and my end.

Saint Teresa of Los Andes

WHY WOMEN?

Traditional female upbringing and sex roles may play a role in the development of women's depression. I remember washing the dishes, biting my lip, as my brothers played baseball outside. I was a better player — the best pitcher in the neighborhood, in fact — and they never had to lift a finger around the house.

According to the National Institute of Mental Health, negative thinking patterns in girls usually develop during those charged teenage years when roles and expectations change quickly and dramatically. During that time, girls are growing breasts, or hoping to, and beginning decades of menstruation. By age fifteen, twice as many girls as boys are likely to have experienced depression. Many more girls than boys will develop eating disorders — starving, abusing, and loathing their new bodies.

In adulthood, women are often poorer than men. More than 75% of those living in poverty in the United States are women and their children. This phenomenon, the feminization of poverty, "may be linked" to depression, says the brochure in my hand. The understatement is almost amusing.

Being single or widowed is a risk factor for depression. And Hispanic women are diagnosed with it more than white women are. African-American women are diagnosed less often, but this may be simply because many of them can't afford health services or because they tend to report physical symptoms rather than the psychological pain they are feeling, leading doctors to overlook what is really wrong. An African-American woman from Georgia once said to me, "It's hard being a black woman. You have to be so strong."

He showed me a little thing about the size of a hazelnut. As I wondered what it could be, the answer came, "It is all that is created." It was so small I wondered how it could survive. In my mind, I heard, "It lasts because God loves it." In this tiny object, I saw three truths: God made it, God loves it, and God takes care of it.

Blessed Julian of Norwich

REPRODUCTIVE EVENTS

I have waded through thousands of words written about depression, going slowly to avoid any danger of being swamped and going slowly because that is all I can manage. As I read, my eyes often turn downwards and I stare at my breasts, my belly, my thighs. My thoughts always return to the female body.

It is women, of course, who have PMS — that unsettling, lonely, psychological turbulence that is followed a few days later by core-deep cramps. It is women who, after pushing babies into the world, sometimes suffer postpartum depression. These new mothers may experience a mild version of depression that has been characterized, and minimized as, "the baby blues." Or they may be driven mad, like the devoted mother who drowns her son or daughter in a bathtub or does some other unspeakable act.

Many women cannot bear children, and given our own expectations and those of others this becomes a terrible burden, badly affecting a woman's sense of self.

I have learned that menopause is not a risk factor for depression. Some women do become depressed during this time of life, but they do so only if they have a history of depression in their family already.

Medical researchers call these things — menstruation, pregnancy, childbirth, infertility, and menopause — "reproductive events." This is such as tepid phrase for things so central to a woman's life.

Our bodies, these creations that keep us breathing and moving through this life, are a source of joy but also of pain. They protect us from harm, but they also can present a real danger to our well being. Women are paradoxes embodied.

*And she is so full of peace that though she press
her flesh, her nerves, her bones, no other thing
comes forth from them than peace.*

Saint Catherine of Genoa

TREATMENT OPTIONS

The authorities — the doctors, the studies, the mental health institutes — assure us that treatment for depression is effective. This is a broad statement, almost too broad to be reliable, almost too general to be true. Our cynical antenna picks up a wave of overconfidence that may or may not be there.

We can't deny the sensible position that treatment works better if it starts earlier. First, we must get a complete physical exam to rule out physical illness as the cause of our depression. Many physical things, especially hypothyroidism, can cause depression. Once the physical causes have been ruled out, we need to get evaluated by a qualified mental-health professional: a psychologist, a psychiatrist, or a clinical social worker.

The most common treatments are either antidepressant medication — generally white or blue pills that make you gain weight — or some form of psychotherapy. In severe cases, ECT (electro-convulsive treatment), might be advised, especially if the depressed patient's life is in danger. Once known as "shock therapy," the mere mention of ECT sends shivers down most people's spines, but the treatment is much improved over the ECT of old. There are also non-traditional (or at least non-Western) treatments such as acupuncture, various forms of meditation, and other therapies that you can try.

Consider yourself a partner in your treatment. Choose a treatment that is right for you. Change treatments or get a second opinion if you are not getting better or if your symptoms worsen. These are nice thoughts but ones that are much easier said than done. The doctor-patient relationship is an unequal one to start with, and who is more powerless than a depressed woman?

Depression is a juggernaut. After diagnosis, we feel as if we are being sucked into a gigantic system of treatment with vacuum-force. Above all, we have to remember to hold on to our true selves.

Our soul is like a castle created out of a single diamond or some other similarly clear crystal.

Saint Teresa of Avila

MEDICATION MISTAKES

It's remarkable that something so insubstantial can turn a life around, but that's what this little pill promises. "It's very effective," the psychiatrist tells me. "Even better," he says, "it has few side effects." This is the case with most of the newer antidepressants.

People taking some of the older, or first generation, pills didn't have it so easy, my doctor says. Anyone taking a group of drugs called the MAO-inhibitors had to avoid some foods, like tofu and smoked fish, and limit their intake of others, such as avocado and chocolate. These foods contain an amino acid that interacted badly with the medication, causing headaches, mania, and other unwanted effects. I shiver slightly when I hear this, feeling thankful to be prescribed a newer drug.

Then a cruel curveball comes my way.

On the second week of taking the new pills, my chest, arms, and back are carpeted in red spots. The rash is not itchy, which is one small mercy, but it has begun creeping up my neck and soon it will be impossible for me to go outside without attracting unwelcome attention.

The psychiatrist's jaw drops when he sees me.

"This is amazing," he says. "You're the second patient in a week to come in with this reaction to this drug."

He turns me around, and I feel like a specimen in a lab. He pushed me gently into a chair and plunks into his own, picking up the telephone receiver. He blabs on, presumably to a colleague. I feel like a freak in a circus.

He hangs up the phone.

"You'll have to try another medication," he announces.

My mouth tightens. Antidepressant drugs often don't take effect for weeks, and now precious time has been lost. I'll have to wait another week before starting a new prescription, since the doctor wants this drug out of my system first.

He hands me another white slip of paper containing the promise of relief. But that has happened before, and I feel my hope seeping away.

Returning to myself, I became depressed and was weary of my life. I almost lacked the patience to go on living.

Blessed Julian of Norwich

COUNSELING THERAPY

The psychiatrist is not unkind. In fact, he means well. He's stiff and seems a little unsure of himself sometimes, but when it's time to end the appointment, he always says, "Hang in there!"

It took years before any other form of treatment besides medication was suggested to me, years before I realized that I needed a different kind of healing than pills can offer. At best, they are not enough for me.

Maggie is my new psychologist; her manner is casual but attentive. She wears an outdated pageboy haircut that gives her the look of the fun-loving young woman she was a few decades ago. Most of her patients are women. Maggie specializes in cognitive-behavioral therapy. It's a mouthful all right, but it is a way of helping a patient change the thought patterns that might be contributing to her problems.

For anyone who is given to lots of thinking and contemplation, as I am, this technique has a great deal of appeal. I can't wait to get started.

As the weeks pass, I learn about cognitive distortions — or unhelpful thinking. Quite simply, Maggie teaches me that if something bad happens, it doesn't mean it's part of a never-ending pattern of defeat. If you feel like a twit, it doesn't mean you are a twit. Instead of saying, "I'm a loser or stupid," it's more appropriate to say, "I made a mistake."

Like many women who have lived with depression for a long time, I discount the positives in my life and dwell on the negatives. I tend to blow little things out of proportion, while serious things, like physical health problems, are ignored or minimized. At some point in my life, I became a black-and-white thinker, but I learn from Maggie that real life is mostly shades of gray.

Maggie imparts wonderful lessons that will carry me through to the end of my days. There's a stack of homework; retraining one's mind is like being a baby learning to walk. But the forest has emerged from the blur of the trees. And I resolve that I am never going down the rocky path of depression alone.

I am the strength and goodness of fatherhood. I am the wisdom of motherhood. I am the light and grace of holy love. I am the Trinity. I am the unity. I teach you to love. I teach you to desire. I am the reward of all true desire.

Blessed Julian of Norwich

TOUGHEN UP

"You can pull yourself out of it if you want," he says.

"It's not that simple."

"Well, it's no way to go through life being down all the time."

"It's not what I want either. I didn't ask for it."

"It's your negative attitude, you've always looked on the down side. Your friend Catherine never does that; she's always smiling and happy."

"Dad, I'm not Catherine. I wish I was, okay, but I'm not."

"I'm just saying that if you smiled more...."

"You're actually saying a lot more than that."

"There's no need to be like that. I'm just trying to help. I've been around a lot longer than you."

"You're lucky you never had to deal with depression. You have no idea what it's like."

"I never had it easy either, you know. I went to bed hungry when I was a kid, we never had anything."

"I know, Dad, I know. I'm sorry."

"You just need to be a little stronger, that's all. Toughen up a bit, change your attitude."

Frozen silence.

"That's the way I see it, Maura."

"I know how you see it, Dad. You never asked me how I see it, though."

Love was His meaning.

Blessed Julian of Norwich

MEMORY

Depression robs us of memory, not in the permanent way that Alzheimer's disease does but more in the way of the forgetfulness of old age.

The mistakes, some of them quite embarrassing, mount up.

It is one of the many minor but undocumented results of the disease.

At a time of such radical change,
it is impossible for nature not to be upset.

Saint Jane de Chantal

THE SNAKE

How dare you, God?
How could you desert me?
Your promises are false.
You have abandoned me, as I suspected you would.
I am alone.
I am without hope.
I have a vicious snake slithering through my brain.

"Where were you
when all of this was happening?"
"I was in your heart."

Saint Catherine of Siena

SUPPORT GROUP

With its gray blockiness, the downtown building was uninviting. The corridors were dusty, the carpet aging and frayed. The words on the little sign outside the room were bald and bold: "Depression Support Group." Cold black ink on lined paper, the kind used by school children the world over. It was crumpled at the bottom, indicating carelessness or rush.

But it was hard to imagine a more impressive group that those who gathered inside, wandering in one by one and taking a place on second-hand folding chairs that would make our bodies numb after only half an hour.

Wynn-Ann had lost her husband and daughter because of the depression that had overcome her. She had spent her way to a lonely life in a boarding house near the waterfront. She relied on the Salvation Army for clothing and for an occasional hot bowl of soup. But she was still breathing, still moving along, still trying.

Darlene had survived twenty-six foster homes. She had blond hair strung down to her shoulders and was Hollywood-actress thin and looked as frail as an eggshell. But she was strong enough to come to the group. And there was a telling firmness in her chin, a hint that she would make it.

Paula spent most of her energy trying to haul herself back to reality, sometimes in a hospital, sometimes at home. But she, too, was still here.

Amy was a teacher with a passion for the children she taught. She deeply loved her family: her loyal, patient husband and her two young daughters. She struggled mightily with the seemingly inexplicable sadness that all but consumed her. But she kept making breakfast for her kids and drawing up lesson plans for her students. She kept coming too.

All of us in the support group were still getting up in the morning, still trying to get through the day, sometimes hour-by-hour and even minute-by-minute. But we were still reaching out to others, those we already knew and to new people. In so doing, we were reaching out to life.

When our group gathered, there were sometimes tears and sometimes sobs. Occasionally, there were unkind remarks. But always, always, there was love. Every time we met, God was among us, an invisible-to-the-eye member of our little group.

Every day I notice that kindness,
gentleness, and support,
as well as generosity,
can do so much for souls.

Saint Jane de Chantal

THE CRY FOR HELP

Maureen told our support group about how, when she was seventeen, she could think of no other plan than to kill herself. She wanted only the darkness and silence that death offered. She said she had been miserable for as long as she could remember, until she met Mark, her high school boyfriend. But a few months into their teenage romance, Mark had told her he had a new girlfriend and that he didn't want to see her anymore.

Maureen said she had stood on the green grass of the high school in a stupor until she snapped out of it and went home. She rushed upstairs and dove at her bed, where she stayed sobbing all night. Her mother brought a tray of sandwiches into her room, telling her, "You've got to eat, Maureen, no matter what's wrong."

The next day, late in the afternoon, Maureen took a sharp shiny knife from the kitchen drawer and went back upstairs. In the bathroom, she cut her wrists and watched the red flow over the white porcelain. An unfamiliar peace came over her.

When she woke up she was in a gleaming white hospital room, covered in a dull green gown. Her mother was sitting in a hard chair near the end of her bed. "Everything will be fine," she said to her foggy-headed daughter.

That was it. Her parents took Maureen home that night, and no one ever spoke of the incident again. It was as if it had never happened.

Accept this spring of tears,
You who empty the seawater from the clouds.
Bend to the pain in my heart, You
whose incarnation bent the sky
and left it empty.

From "Troparion,"
a hymn sung on Holy Tuesday
by Saint Kassiane

THE SECRET

I got talking to a woman I met at a conference in New Mexico, and it turned out we had something in common. Deshanté never said a word to anyone about how she felt. She dragged herself out of bed and through each day, filled with fear and a corrosive sadness. She was twenty-four before she talked about her feelings to any one, but she had lived with them since her early teens.

Deshanté felt she had to keep quiet about her depression, but she was never sure why. Perhaps she was afraid no one would understand, or that they might make a joke of her misery. Maybe she feared her few friends might blow her off or her parents might tell her not to be so melodramatic. Early on she decided that they'd dismiss her low moods as a teenage phase. But it was a phase that didn't lift, no matter what she did.

So Deshanté kept quiet, plodding through the days, weeks, months, and years. This was her life — no more, no less.

She was certain she was the only one who felt this way. After all, everyone else seemed happy. There were, it seemed, smiles wherever she looked, except when she looked in the mirror. The person she saw there — the young woman with stringy brown hair and glassy eyes — was the only one who knew the secret of her illness, until she began sharing her story.

You who want
knowledge,
seek the Oneness
within
There you
will find
the clear mirror
already waiting

Hadewijch of Antwerp

BURDEN

Sarah is one of the quietest members of the support group. She's tiny and birdlike and it's hard not to worry about her. She studies graphic arts at a local community college but has had to postpone exams because of her depression. Tears sit on her eyelids as she talks about falling further behind.

Then she spills out her greatest fear. Sarah is lonely and wants a boyfriend. She's only twenty and thinks that if she doesn't get a guy soon she never will. There are a couple of young men at the college who are cute, she says, and one of them sits next to her in class and has introduced himself. But she is afraid to let go and seek out his company.

"I'd have to tell him about my depression," she explains. "And then what would he say? He'd think I'm crazy or just walk away, and then I'd feel like an idiot."

We all tried to encourage her to take a chance, at least when she was ready. Forgetting our own afflictions, we wanted all good things for her. But Sarah didn't have the strength to risk it, at least not yet.

The forget-me-not asks Him
*   for a stronger brilliance*
in her blue eyes
and the ant asks Him for more strength
to grip the straw.
And the bees ask Him for a stronger victory song
among scarlet roses.

Edith Södergran

RUNNING AWAY

Olivia could not take another diaper change, another potato to peel, another strained conversation with a husband she loved but didn't want around anymore. She couldn't stand to open any of the books that were taking her towards an M.B.A. She wanted to hide under her bedcovers and stay there until death claimed her. She was neither hungry nor thirsty. She felt nothing but a quiet desperation.

Her cousin had a cabin in the Michigan woods, and one day Olivia went there. She left her children asleep in their beds, knowing their father was on his way home, and off she went, more than 100 miles away.

She knew where her cousin kept the key and reached behind the window frame and pulled it out. She knew people would condemn her for running away, but she had to leave.

"I was saving my life," she told our support group.

Olivia was right. Her days in the silent woods reminded her of the strengths she had that she could draw upon. On the second day away, she phoned her husband, who told her he was glad she was safe. She told him she loved him.

Finally, she returned home. Her husband pulled her into a giant bear hug, along with their kids.

At first, Olivia could hardly face the drudgery of her life again, but her running away had cemented something important in her, as well as in her relationship with her husband and children.

If I desire something, I know it not,
For in a boundless of unknowing
I have lost my very self.
In His mouth I am engulfed,
In a bottomless abyss;
Never could I come out of it.

Hadewijch of Antwerp

REMEMBERING

A therapist once asked me to recall a happy memory from my childhood. For a long time silence filled the room.

Finally, I saw myself in a department store cafeteria with my mother. I was eating French fries followed by ice cream, grinning all the while.

I remembered that I had been having a difficult time at school at the time and had been slapped by teacher (a nun who I eventually came to understand was very troubled). In that store, with my mother, on that day, only safety and protection surrounded me.

I did not want the lunch to end.

A land not mine, still
forever memorable,
the waters of its ocean
chill and fresh.

Anna Akhmatova

PERFECTION

When you are depressed, everyone else's life looks perfect. You are the only one who is not a member of the Walton clan or the Brady Bunch — big caring families who always seem to solve their problems with love and respect. These were TV families, of course, but we all know real families who resemble them (or at least seem to from the outside). It seems that we are the only ones with problems and struggles.

The reality, of course, is quite different. No one, literally, is perfect, and bad things do happen to good people all the time.

These lessons are given to us over and over. But we find it hard to remember them if we are depressed.

*Abandon all your desires for advancement
and perfection; hand them over completely into
God's hands. Leave the care of them to Him.*

Saint Jane de Chantal

ABANDONMENT

Abandonment is like being stuck in a narrow well that reaches into the freezing bowels of the earth. This is the worst aspect of depression for me. Like a hungry bear, it threatens and endangers me.

They say the fear of abandonment is a temporary problem. But who, under its powerful thumb, can believe that? It's too big; its heft is too substantial. And I am small, weak, and helpless.

Right now words like "permanent" and "temporary" have no meaning. At times like this, the only solution for me is to disappear to a place where there can be no more hurt, because there is no more feeling.

Woe is me, your mother, woe is me,
your daughter — why have you abandoned me
like an orphan?

Blessed Hildegard of Bingen
(writing to her friend Richardis)

STAYING

Still here.
Weary and wounded.
But still here.
That is all I can be for now.

The weaker she becomes,
the greater are the miracles she works
according to her strength
with his power.

Mechtild of Magdeburg

MUSIC

Few of us listen to music anymore. I mean really listen: just sitting there — not reading or cooking or talking or eating — but just listening to music.

It's easy to be romantic about a less technologically advanced time, but it is true that people once had the solace of music, uncluttered by a thousand distractions.

A woman living with depression can listen to music without expending too much psychic energy. It doesn't matter if we listen to Fearon, Loretta Lynn, Billie Holiday, or Christina Aguilera. Or bluegrass, country, classical, or salsa. Even Blessed Hildegard's music now reaches to us from across the centuries. We can hear the lyrics and melodies birthed by medieval women.

Music is one way to be with God and perhaps experience some respite.

God placed high spiritual delight in my soul. I was completely filled with confidence, and resolutely sustained. I dreaded nothing. It was such a happy spiritual feeling that I was totally at peace. Nothing on earth could have disturbed me.

Blessed Julian of Norwich

SELF-RECRIMINATION

Not for the first time, I've snapped at my husband. It's me, not him. I know that. He knows that. My patience has all but deserted me. My body is like something hit by lightening: frantic, nervous, jumpy. I feel like I am teetering on the edge of a cliff.

Paul has not lost his patience. His massive ability to give love endures. He amazes me.

When a little calm is restored, we talk about it. I feel terrible; no one has loved or supported me more than him.

There have been times he's snapped at me, he says. He's not perfect, he reminds me.

"Thank, God." I say. "If you were, you'd show me up something awful."

We end up laughing and hugging, my depression receding into the night.

When you find yourself committing one fault or another, just humble yourself quietly before God by a simple acknowledgment of the fault and think no more about it.

Saint Jane de Chantal

PLEASING OTHERS

From the day we leave the womb, girls and women are expected to please: our parents, our teachers, our husbands, our partners, our children, our co-workers, our friends. We want to be "good girls," to do as we're told, so that we will be valued. It seems that being female is all about meeting the needs of others.

All over the world, women's duties are extensive. We are the caretakers: of families, of communities, of the sick and the needy. "I don't count anymore," my friend Donna said after she gave birth to her second child twenty years ago. Her words were shocking but also truthful and memorable.

With the burden of responsibilities so many of us women have, it is not easy to take such time. Sometimes — and even for years on end — it's only the top priorities in our lives that get our attention.

Sometimes we pretend we are not as smart as we are really are. Other times we agree with someone even though we are opposed to or even offended by what they are saying. Before long, such self-deprecation can become a habit. Because of some pretty twisted expectations, we end up not being ourselves. We forget who we are, what we feel, what we think.

Maybe there is a link to women's depression in all this.

My self-confidence depends on the fact that I have discovered my dimensions. It does not become me to make myself less than I am.

Edith Södergran

CRASHING

Angela made lunches for her two kids every night. She washed and dried their clothes as they slept. She prepared oatmeal for their breakfasts, and poured orange juice into glasses so that they'd have their Vitamin C. She helped them gather their backpacks and put their coats on in the fall and winter and drove them to school.

Sometimes she slept when her husband and kids were gone in the day. She had to; she collapsed into the bed or, when she was too tired to go to her bedroom, on the sofa. She never told her husband Peter about these naps. She didn't want him to think she was lazy.

Every week, Angela counted down the days to the weekend. On Saturdays she permitted herself to stay in bed, the only place she didn't feel overwhelmed and exhausted. Peter took the kids to Little League or the mall. She didn't care where they went.

Thus does depression sap every once of energy we have.

*The Spirit of God
is a life that bestows life,
root of world-tree
and wind in its boughs.*

*Scrubbing out sin,
she rubs oil into wounds.*

*She is glistening life
alluring all praise,
all-awakening,
all resurrecting.*

Blessed Hildegard of Bingen

PRAYER
of the
DEPRESSED

Clara was a deeply religious woman, going to Mass daily whenever she could, saying the rosary every night, just as her late mother had taught her to do in childhood. Clara graduated from college and taught elementary school. She married Don, a real estate agent, and had two daughters, who were now grown. She was looking forward to retiring from teaching and pursuing her watercolor painting.

Then, suddenly, in mid-life, depression hit Clara like a piece of granite. She felt like another person, a ghost in place of herself. "It's like I don't know where I am most of the time," she explained, her eyes wide with the shock of what was happening to her. "It's like I can't find myself."

Clara had always turned to prayer when trouble hit her — when her mother died, when she didn't get tenure at her first school — and it never failed to wrap her in comfort. But now prayer deserted her. She couldn't engage in prayer or even try. Prayer had become a foreign language to her. She was horrified and frightened. "I feel naked," she said, biting her stubby fingernails. "And I'm letting God down by not praying. I'm not doing my duty."

Clara went to a wise nun for spiritual mentoring. The nun told her that God was patient with the sick and wanted nothing from Clara. The nun taught her to sit with God, not worrying about prayer, not saying anything. Clara could do this and began taking baby steps in her new relationship with God.

Simply the presence of our spirit before His and His before ours forms prayer, whether or not we have fine thoughts or feelings.

Saint Jane de Chantal

SELF-PITY

Why me? What did I do to deserve this intractable depression?

The "why me's?" cover me like a bad rash. They itch and scratch and drive me to distraction. They forbid banishment. They offer only temptation to wallow in them.

Meanwhile the newspapers are full of obituaries of people who have died of cancer who were, apparently, all brave and courageous. But is this true? Or did they lie there afraid to say how they really felt, closed in by the white-washed hospital walls, in pain and in grief facing the greatest fear of them all, the one we all share. Did they really swallow their hurt, worry, and uncertainty?

We're in a stiff upper lip society. In some ways, our Christian faith glorifies suffering. We're told it makes us better people, brings us closer to God. "If it doesn't kill you, it makes you stronger," we tell one another.

For those of us who are depressed, however, these messages ring in our ears at a time when it is hard to hear them. For us, the "why me's?" have the sharp edge of broken glass piercing soft flesh.

But I and those who loved me wondered why such great persecution came upon me, and why God did not bring me comfort.

Blessed Hildegard of Bingen

SELF-LOATHING

The kernel of self-loathing that usually lies buried within my heart now rises to the surface. Like a hungry wolf under the night sky, it howls, its cries cutting through the air.

My body appears ugly, even deformed, to me.

"Are you anorexic?" asks the counselor, a jocular, heavy, motherly lady who is forever offering me chocolate chip cookies and cups of tea. I'm not, I assure her; I love chicken breasts, gooey pizza, and buttery croissants too much for that, even now. But, like those women who cannot bring life-giving food to their pinched lips, I've begun to hate my body. And my body, of course, is myself.

I cannot hear when the man who loves me tells me I'm beautiful. He is speaking a tongue I have no hope of deciphering. If he could hear the responses in my head he wouldn't even bother trying.

At night I obsess about how my father never once said I was pretty. A relentlessly recurring image is of my friend Lisa's father telling her how lucky he is to have such a pretty daughter. The man's words assault my ears, like pointed fingernails on a black board. A sense of deprivation fuels my anger, but the anger quickly dissipates, like a mist evaporating. It transforms itself into despair and a tornado of tears.

I desired you before the world began.
I desire you now
As you desire me.

Mechtild of Magdeburg

WHAT TO DO?

A depressed woman does not put much effort into her social life. Yet invitations to lunch, dinner, or a quick coffee at the corner still trickle in. They take the form of a friendly email or a message left on the phone. Even reading or listening to them is threatening.

But, in spite of the bear-like urge to hibernate, there is another, smaller wish: To say, "Yes, I'd love to go, I'll be there."

Planning has become impossible, though. Who can tell which days will be good and which will be crushingly difficult? How tolerable will the company of another person be when we get there? Will there be enough energy to summon the required happy face? For how long? There is no predicting it, and so it is safer to say "no."

Depression makes clear that the world is, above all, social. Friendship and all manner of gatherings are celebrated. Extroverts are lauded and applauded. Introverts are treated with suspicion. (Meanwhile, depression makes introverts of everyone it grips.)

Being women, however, we don't want to give offence, and saying "no" might offend. Nor do we want to lose the life-saving safety rope that companionship offers. Deep down, we want out of the swamp of our depression, but invitations result in terror-fueled adrenalin rushes and twisting innards. What to do? What to do? What to do?

*Pain rises up within me. Pain kills the great trust
and the solace that I found in a human being.*

Blessed Hildegard of Bingen

SUFFERING

"God gave you this depression for a reason," the older woman said.

"I don't see why God would do that," the younger woman answered.

"That's the way God works."

"You think God is a puppet master, up there pulling strings? You think God sat there on a cloud one day and decided to inflict me with depression, of all things?"

The older woman paused. "He only does it for a good reason. You should offer it up as a sacrifice for people who need God's help."

"I need God's help, and I need it now. This is all so superstitious."

"It's not. Everyone knows that suffering is good for the soul. It purifies us."

"If we survive it! Why are people so judgmental about illness?"

"It's not judgment, it's faith. If you carry the cross, it will carry you. That's what Saint Thomas à Kempis said."

Now the younger woman hesitated. "You're on to something," she said, "but I don't really understand it. The saints tried to make sense of suffering and saw it as multi-dimensional. They tried to give it meaning. Saint Augustine said suffering is medicine, but even he said that God was a physician and that sickness was not a punishment."

"Maybe it is more complicated than I thought. Just remember that God is with you in your suffering. You're a child of God."

"I am, whether I suffer or not."

*God has nowhere to put his goodness, if not in
me, no place to put himself entire, if not in me.
And by this means I am the exemplar of salvation,
and what is more, I am the salvation itself of every
creature, and the glory of God.*

Marguerite Porete

FAULT

"Maybe this depression happened so you would learn empathy," the priest says, a fleck of judgment in his ice-blue eyes. He doesn't have a clue. I don't need to learn empathy, I tell him, surprising myself with a sudden rush of insight and confidence. I am already sensitive to the needs of others, both stated and unstated. In fact, if this were not so, my depression might not be so intense. Maybe I would be better at looking after myself more effectively if empathy for others was not such a constant companion.

The priest is taken aback and says nothing. Does he realize that he has been presumptuous about someone he hardly knows (and something he probably doesn't understand, unless he too suffers from depression)? Or does he merely think that the young woman in front of him is arrogant and selfish?

Everything happens for a reason, he says. But beneath all the guilt and superstition that this notion represents, there is in us women who suffer from depression a dim awareness that we have not been selected for this particular form of suffering. There is no god up there trying to teach us bitter lessons. We aren't pawns. There is no giant chessboard. There is no one keeping track of all we do and devising ways of making sure we do things his way or else.

Everything does not happen for a reason. There is chaos through the universe. We don't always cause what happens to us. We did nothing to deserve this. We are not to blame.

We have to remember this, above all else.

His left hand, in heat of noonday,
Lovingly my head upholds,
And his right hand, filled with blessings,
Tenderly my soul enfolds.

Ann Griffiths

WHAT HAPPENED, HAPPENED

It is easy to forget or dismiss our own problems. Difficult to remember that we have a right to feel sad or blue...or even desperate or chilled with fear. It is so easy to scrub out our own history, so tempting to minimize the steep hills and low valleys of our own life.

"It was nothing," we say, but the things that have happened to us cannot really be dismissed so easily. We may think they are all over, that they happened so long ago, that they didn't bother us that much, that we're over them now. "Worse things have happened to other people," we say to ourselves.

But perhaps it's not that simple. Perhaps the pain and hurt still chafes and digs. Maybe it pokes our souls, shoving sticks into our peace of mind.

What happened to us may be big or small in the scheme of things. It might have happened once; it might have happened a hundred times. But what happened to us mattered.

Regardless of what happens, be gentle with yourself.

Saint Jane de Chantal

THE SPIRIT ON THE RADIO

The old pop song "Spirit in the Sky" blasts from the car radio. The song combines a simple but comforting and celebratory theology with bouncy, happy music.

> Never been a sinner, I never sinned
> I got a friend in Jesus
> So you know that when I die
> He's gonna set me up with
> The Spirit in the Sky.

Hearing this song is as refreshing as a cold shower on a sweltering day. It's enough to lift my depression. Music can do that.

You are my Father and my God
for whom I expect all my happiness.

Saint Jane de Chantal

LIMPING ALONG

Everyone in the depression support group is ailing or can vividly recall ailments that accompany their episodes of depression. Wynn-Ann has terrible headaches that force her to stay in light- and sound-free rooms, sometimes for days at a time. Rose is laid low by constant stomach pains. They've both been through myriad medical tests with no diagnoses resulting. Their physical pains are as mysterious as their mental anguish.

And I, never having broken a bone in my life and never having had my muscles challenged by zealous participation in sports, have suddenly developed a limp. It seems to originate somewhere from the region of my right knee, but the odd, persistent feeling there is too general to call "pain." Yet the avoidance of the kind of hard floors in shopping malls and other places has become necessary. It's not significant enough to warrant a visit to the doctor, much less the hospital emergency. But it's significant enough that it's like a constant conversation with the volume not quite high enough to make out what is being said.

Most of us in the support group are in our thirties and forties so we make all kinds of jokes about deciding which senior citizens' home we are going to check into. The best-looking staff is at Saint Joseph's, Wynn-Ann says.

"It's all in my head!" she adds, and the room fills with laughter, keeping our collective depression at bay for one precious moment.

And, try, for the love of God, to restore your former strength by getting enough rest, physically and mentally, and by taking plenty of good, nourishing food.

Saint Jane de Chantal

THE TUG OF WAR

Over and over, I second-guess myself. I don't allow myself to feel what something in me wants desperately to feel: sadness; deep loneliness; anxiety. The list goes on and grows.

There's self-admonishment too: All this is self-pity and I've got no right to it. Some of the things that cause daggers in my heart are hardly tragedies or disasters but only pettiness and nonsense.

I won't let myself mourn anything, even the losses that linger. I am like a knight guarding a fortress. I'm trying to keep myself together by keeping myself away from harm; yet the most threatening harm, it seems, comes from inside me.

I won't give myself permission to do the necessary reflection and expression. I expend a fair amount of energy punching and slapping my mind and heart into reluctant submission. This tug of war drains whatever sparks I have left. Deep down I know I am imperiling myself, but there is nothing to stop me and no one to help, because I keep all these things buried deep inside.

I have thought myself into emptiness.

Let nothing disturb thee,
Nothing affright thee;
All things are passing;
God never changeth.

Saint Teresa of Avila

ASSERTING MYSELF

God knows asserting ourselves doesn't come easy for most depressed women, including me. The notion inevitably rises to the surface that assertive women are unattractive or worse, and I don't want to be viewed that way. It's against the instincts that have been embedded in my very marrow: no one will like me; everyone will leave me.

But I try. I summon courage to tell my boss his actions are not acceptable, not in this case, not in this way. It works. After a moment's hesitation, he backs off. My chest puffs up with a heady combination of relief and pride.

It doesn't always work, of course. Sometimes the price is too high. Conflict, I come to realize, is part of the natural order of things. It need not be so threatening. It won't always lead to disaster.

God placed high spiritual delight in my soul. I was completely filled with confidence, and resolutely sustained. I dreaded nothing. It was such a happy spiritual feeling that I was totally at peace. Nothing on earth could have disturbed me.

Blessed Julian of Norwich

SILVER LEAVES

The little tree is only a foot high, and its width is just as modest. It's almost a shrub — is there really an adult tree in there waiting to burst out? The trunk is nearly as thin as a straw, but it's a rich burgundy, boasting health and potential. We plant it near the house, affording our new friend some shelter from the fierce northeasterly winds that frequently blow this way.

Our new tree is a silver leaf dogwood. As it takes root, I can feel layers of depression inexplicably peeling themselves away. I'm a snake shaking off old skin.

The new tree still resembles a bush by the end of our short summer. But the next year it grows more than a foot. Another fall arrives, followed by an unending winter. The tree jumps to life in the tentative spring sunshine and grows two feet in July and August.

It is now taller than I am, its leaves a neat pea-green lined with a gentle yellow. It's as wide as a barrel, its long branches saluting the big sky all around.

My friend, it is impossible to stand next to you without smiling and feeling a rush of love and hope.

Thou art a very daughter to me, and a mother also,
a sister, a wife and a spouse.

Margery Kempe

THE LIZARD

Depression has rendered me an orphan.

When I was a child I knew that God loved me. Now, despite a pressing need to feel the divine presence and a longing to feel divine love, God remains elusive.

Mostly the lizard that is my brain dominates. It directs me to eat enough potatoes and drink enough orange juice to stay alive, but intelligent thought is largely suspended.

Someday, I tell myself, God will wrap me in her arms and pour her mother's love on me.

This much I know is true.

And feeling such pain from Him, I felt myself totally aflame with the most sweet love of this most sweet Lord. Little by little, He lifted me up on high, thus uniting Himself to this, my unworthy body.

Maria Domitilla Galluzzi

LOOKING FOR GOD

Louisa was frantic to find God; desperation had taken over her very soul. She went to Mass but could not hear the words through the fog of depression she now lived in. She went on a guided nature walk, peering into the bushes at the furtive little catbirds, but they signified nothing. She chanted with Shambhala Buddhists, willing God to come to her but nothing did.

She told herself that at least God would appreciate her long, continuing search. She realized that, deep down, she believed that God would cure her depression if only she could restore that severed link.

Then a liberating thought hit Louisa. Its obviousness made her laugh: God is not a thing to be found in one place. God is absolutely everywhere, all the time.

The day of my spiritual awakening was the day I saw and knew I saw all things in God and God in all things.

Mechtild of Madgeburg

VISION

Saint Francis de Sales once said that God gives us suffering that is "not one inch too long and not one ounce too heavy." Spiritual bromides similar to this are well-known to most of us.

But they are not true! Psychiatric wards are full of people who could just not take it anymore; young men and women see no other option but to put an end to their pain by cutting their wrists or putting a handgun in their mouth; and millions see mind-altering drugs and alcohol as their only hope of dealing with their demons. Clearly, some of us have been on the receiving end of suffering that is indeed too long and too heavy.

There are many such untruths engrained in us, many from our Judeo-Christian heritage. Sometimes these lies are hurtful and damaging.

Many Christians believe that those who are disabled or are carrying one cross or another are favored, even chosen or loved specially, by God. At first, this notion might seem to offer a sense of comfort, a kind of compensation for the pain that claws at the sufferer's heart, body, or mind.

But it's not true either. Nor is the longstanding idea that God tests us through illness, accidents, and other calamities and then rewards us for putting up with them, preferably without complaint.

In a very odd way, depression brings with it a new, liberating clarity. As the depressed person moves through it, she can see what is true and what isn't, what is real and what isn't. Everything else, the myriad clutter, is stripped away. With depression smothering one's very being, every thought and idea that makes it through to our brain is of more consequence than usual. Everything is put in sharp relief. There are meaningful lessons and then healing in this.

What God, in His goodness, asks of you is a calm, peaceful uselessness, a resting near Him with no special attention or action of the understanding or will except a few words of love, or of faithful, simple surrender, spoken softly, effortlessly, without the least desire to find consolation or satisfaction in them. If you put that into practice, I will promise you, it will please God more than anything else you might do.

Saint Jane de Chantal

HONING MY ACTING SKILLS

Any woman who has ever suffered from depression could win an Academy Award for acting. Kate Winslset, Marion Cotillard, Helen Mirren, Reese Witherspoon, Hilary Swank, Charlize Theron, Nicole Kidman, Halle Berry, and Julia Roberts all could take lessons from us.

As a depressed woman goes through the motions, her innate acting skills emerge, take shape, and develop. She smiles when she feels a monkey wrench twisting away in her tummy. She chats with friends when she'd rather be carried away by sleep. When she can, she shows up at the office or for class. She fetches a glass of apple juice for her toddler. She listens intently with care to her partner's stories at the end of the day.

But if you asked her, she will admit that it is often an act. One of the worst parts of depression is the every-present feeling that you are a fraud, that whenever you are not alone you are acting to please others. There is the real you and the public you, the latter leeching energy from the former.

Yet, as we go about our acting career, it is worth remembering that much of the time something is holding us up, allowing us to deliver our next line. What could that possibly be?

The more silent she remains, the louder she cries.

Mechtild of Madgeburg

WOMAN-CARE

It would be wonderful to have perfect mental health. But many of us do not. Some of us will have to live with depression or the threat of depression for many years, if not all our lives.

Depression may well be one of the worst illnesses a human being can experience. It is certainly one of the most complex and misunderstood, even to those of us who live with it.

Perhaps, like all illnesses, depression can teaches us to take better care of ourselves, first and foremost. As women, this may be the first time we have ever been called upon to take care of ourselves. The trick is to get a workable balance between hyper-vigilance and complete disregard. There is a lot of room in the middle between these two.

So, having given you a delicate constitution, He expects you to take care of it and not demand of it what He Himself, in his gentleness, does not ask for. Accept this fact.

Saint Jane de Chantal

ADVICE

The plastic hospital bracelet leaves my wrist a little tender. The soreness is still there when I return to work. Dick, a fellow academic I don't know well, greets me in the hallway.

"How are you? You look tired, but I hope you're feeling better."

"I'm not too bad, thanks."

"What's your diet like? That might be your problem."

"My diet's normal, it's okay."

"You ought to take vitamin supplements, maybe you've got a shortage of Vitamin C. You should drink more orange juice. Cranberry juice is good for your system too."

"Okay. Thanks."

"There's no reason for you to be ill. You'd see a big improvement if you took hold of your diet."

"Well, it's a bit more complicated than that."

For the first time he looks right into my eyes. He can see the resentment that is gathering to a boil. "Yeah. Okay, well, see you around." And he's gone, scurrying down the hall, his knapsack bouncing off his back.

And just as we plunge pure wool
In the scarlet dye again and again,
To brighten and fix the color,
God transforms and guides the soul:
Difficulty and plunging grief
Will deepen its hue and its worth.
And if for love of your Creator
You can find patience in this sorrow,
You will surely receive highest gift —
You will walk in glory and honor,
In the vision of the Savior,
Having lived and burned for Him in human flesh.

The French Beguine

DULLNESS

Saint John of the Cross made the phrase, "the dark night of the soul," hauntingly familiar. It is often used to describe depression — or at least certain forms or phases of it.

Sometimes depression is not crushingly oppressive. Sometimes it does not plunge you into a pit of despair. Sometimes it does not make us want to yell or screech or shout.

Sometimes there is just the feeling that we are encased in numbness as if slowly emerging from anesthetic. We feel nothing. We can hardly speak. Words fly by our ears instead of entering them. Putting one foot in front of the other seems impossible. Fatigue is part of it, but there is much more than that going on, even though it appears there is absolutely nothing happening at all.

Psychiatrists call this odd state "lack of affect." Anyone experiencing it feels like a dull knife, a worn-out dirty sock. There's no drama when we are trapped in this cruel dullness, just a dreary hollow echo of nothing.

The dark night of the soul
Is a gray pedestrian place which,
In its very bleakness,
Slowly eats at passion
And vitality.

Edwina Gateley

HELPING OTHERS

A woman's world is made smaller by depression. Sometimes it is tiny to the point of claustrophobia, seeming to be no more than a closet with no door or window.

Christianity teaches us about the value of serving others. We hear about Jesus giving health to the woman who bled and forgiveness and hope to the woman who had committed adultery.

What can we do to help others? How can we emerge from the fogginess of depression to be of use to anyone?

Deep down, we know that helping others will help us — as sick as we are. At least one depressed woman's life was saved through service to others, this I know. It was mine.

Every morning, men in our city roll up their sleeping bags along the city's embankment and make their way to St. Martin's-in-the-Fields to a day center for the homeless located in the ancient, historical crypts. The disheveled dozens come in hungry for a cheese sandwich or itching for a hot shower.

One man, only in his thirties, had lost his job and his wife had left him. Another was an immigrant who couldn't quite get a foothold in his new land. A third had survived the Dachau concentration camp, not whole but still alive.

We volunteers made them tea and helped them fill out housing applications. They gave us an opportunity to come face to face with God.

As I served these men, somehow the torture of my own soul disappeared. Through the act of spreading butter on bread and putting it on a plate for the men, I discovered that — at least for a time — my worries, fears, and troubles were gone.

In order to have peace,
one must forget about oneself.

Saint Elizabeth of the Trinity

FALLING OFF THE WAGON

Lisa tells the other patients in the waiting room that she has "fallen off the old wagon," as she puts it. Gin has been her drug of choice, her way of stumbling through her depression intact. After a year's faithfulness to Alcoholics Anonymous, she had won her one-year sobriety pin.

But now her life was again in tatters and her face was soaked in tears. An unexpected visit from her mother had sent her to that familiar shelf in the store. Her drinking had lasted one night and one day, and then it was over. But Lisa was using words to beat herself up for her transgression. She was, she said, "useless," "stupid," "a loser," "a failure." She went on and on.

Some of us have seen Lisa here before, and now we offer words of encouragement, but these seemed to plunge her further into her obsessive self-recrimination. There seems to be nothing we can do, except hope the doctor can help. Lisa was on the path to self-destruction, and her determination to get there was such that there seemed to be no question of her going anywhere else.

Sometimes there is not a happy ending to the Story of Depression.

When you weep and mourn for My pain and My passion, then you are a very mother having compassion on her child. When you weep for other people's sins and adversities, then you are a very sister.

Margery Kempe

THE SEAMSTRESS

I like being a seamstress. Bits of cloth and long pieces of thread lay on the floor, ready to be joined. The cloth is torn and needs mending. It has a rip and is missing a button or two.

Sewing helps me move at a snail's pace out of depression. I am both the cloth and the seamstress. Both are fragmented and tattered. The seamstress is the one who has to sew the pieces back together, making sure they can't be ripped asunder again. No one else can do it but me. Not even my caring friends or my husband, who long to cure me.

I can't rely on someone else to do the fixing. Ultimately I am completely alone with my depression — at least it feels that way — and I have to put myself back together.

For those of us who suffer from depression, bits of us have died. Maybe we will never be as joyful as we were before this earth-shattering illness descended on us. Perhaps we've grown cynical as family members and friends drifted away or weren't there for us to start with. We come out of this as new women. We might resemble the women who went into depression, but we aren't those women anymore; we're different now, like a tattered dress that has been re-sewn.

What will remain? What should remain? What do we need to let go of? How do we put ourselves back together? Only the seamstress knows.

As certainly as God is our father, just as certainly he is our mother. In our father, we have our being; in our mother, we are remade and restored, our fragmented lives are knit together and made perfect.

Blessed Julian of Norwich

STRUGGLING

My friend Leslie points out that women with depression are in a constant struggle. We tell ourselves we shouldn't feel this way. We try to change our natures as well as our disease. But, of course, this proves impossible most of the time.

In North America we use military imagery when we talk of disease: we "fight" illness, we "battle" cancer, we are "at war" with diabetes.

"I mean, how healthy is that?" Leslie asks. "To think of ourselves in a constant battle. We're sick, it shouldn't be like we're in a war."

She's right. We lose a battle or we win it. But that isn't really this way with an illness, especially a chronic, insidious illness like depression. We're not in a battle; we're on a journey. It might be an extremely challenging and sometimes harrowing journey, but it is a journey nonetheless.

How can an ill person be at war with herself and with her own body? Her illness is part of her. She might even be able to learn from it.

Leslie and I decide to resign from the military and lay down our armor. From now on, we will try to see depression as a journey, not an enemy to be defeated. We determine that we are going to stop struggling to "win" and begin instead to think of depression as something we will live with.

Resign yourself to not being able to resign yourself as completely and utterly as you would like, or as you think our Lord would like.

Saint Jane de Chantal

ANGELS

The unexpected flow of tears is not unknown to women living with depression. But sometimes it's the kindness of others that crashes through our fragile defenses and makes us break down. Those crying jags are different from the others. More hopeful. More thankful. More cleansing.

The pharmacist had crystal blue eyes surrounded by smile lines. His hands were large and moved slowly. He filled the small plastic container with tiny yellow pills. Then he leaned over, his elbows firm on the counter, and looked right into my eyes. In a voice as soft and sweet as cotton candy, he said, "You're going through a very hard time, but you won't always feel this way."

He was my instant guardian angel, an emissary from a loving God, a fellow-resident of a universe in which there is much kindness. As I felt the wetness of tears on my cheeks, my heart swelled.

Your words have kindled me as if a flame would have touched my heart.

Saint Elisabeth of Schönau
(writing to Blessed Hildegard of Bingen)

THE PROMISE

"Will I ever get better?" My eyes are swollen shut from crying.

My husband, Paul, reaches over and pulls me to him. "You will," he whispers, "I know you will."

"Really?" For a minute, I glimpse recovery; it is almost too good to be true.

"Really," he says.

"How do you know?"

He smiles, his eyes soft and gentle. "I know. I just know."

And you would come back to the soul,
To fill her with your blessedness.
There the soul dwells —
Like the fish in the sea
And the sea in the fish.

Saint Catherine of Siena

A CHANGED LIFE

In the hospital one of the nurses told me her story. She had been a nurse for twelve years when her mania struck. She spent every cent she had ever saved, buying a car she didn't need and fur coats she would never wear, and then she crashed, sleeping for four straight days. When she awoke, she cut herself to pieces in an unsuccessful attempt to end her life.

Sabine is bi-polar, afflicted with a challenging disease once known as "manic-depression." She spent six weeks in hospital, tending to her physical and psychic wounds. Fortunately, she responded well to the lithium that her doctors prescribed.

But she had to put her life back together. She could not return to the demanding profession of nursing. Her boyfriend was gone, after saying that Sabine was "too much to handle."

Sabine the nurse had become Sabine the patient. She had to learn to receive care, and she would be in this situation for the rest of her life. With a smile on her face and a twinkle in her eyes, she began to put her life back together, one day at a time.

Therefore, help her so that her vineyard
might not be destroyed.

Blessed Hildegard of Bingen

GOD'S CARE

The thundering noise of the snowmobile tore through the languid silence of the tundra. We drove through dark thickets of stunted black spruce. We skidded over hard-packed snow and icy tracks left by other travelers on this lovely, lonely northern coast of Canada. The snowmobile pushed itself over a ridge as white as dove's feathers, and we halted. The valley below was a bright ivory. In the distance, the silhouettes of a family of caribou darkened the far sky. All was perfectly still now.

A petite snow bunting in black and white winter plumage hopped from one low spruce branch to another. Amazingly, the little bird was completely impervious to the frigid air. She seemed to neither see nor feel the ice crystals that hung in the air like glassy Christmas decorations.

The land beneath us was the bosom of God, and we were being cradled with the purest love, babies at a warm welcoming breast. Even in my depression, I could feel it.

Effortlessly,
Love flows from God into man,
Like a bird
Who rivers the air
Without moving her wings.

Mechtild of Magdeburg

FORGETTING

There comes a time when the tempest ceases and the arctic soul springs again to life. When this happens, the mind stops its bloodletting ,and scabs begin to grow over wounds that were previously open to the air.

Now tomatoes burst in the mouth, sending a sweet wetness over the tongue. The sounds of a child's voice ring clearly in the ears, and it is welcome. The hand relishes again the feel of the stubbly skin of a husband's unshaven cheek. Scarlet is its rich self once more, and blue is comfortingly in all its hues: indigo, royal, baby.

Veins have thawed out, and life-giving blood streams through the body once more. You jump, run, yell, eat, drink. You flop onto a couch, belly-filled and smiling.

Best of all, the dreary hours, days, weeks, months of your latest episode are forgotten. It is almost impossible to recall how slowly and viciously they went by. Memories recede and life lovingly calls you back to itself.

No, you are not "cured." You are, at best, in remission. You will have to live with your depression for the rest of your life. But you are allowed to enjoy this moment.

Live gladly and gaily because of His Love.

Blessed Julian of Norwich

SAFETY

God's love for me is a fleece blanket, enveloping me
and keeping me warm on a crisp December night.
God's love for me is warm water flowing over my body.
God's love for me is the gentle May sun on my face.
God's love for me was there when I was nothing more
than two miniscule cells knitting themselves together.
God's love for me is here now as gray hair sprouts
from my temples.
I belong to God. I can feel it.
Even my depression cannot destroy that feeling of safety.

*I belong to God. He created me
and is my beginning and my end.*

Saint Teresa of Los Andes

REGRETS

A woman who has survived depression is inevitably filled with regret. Her heart is like the hold of a fishing boat, topped to the gunnels with fish.

There is a shopping list of things she could have done: taken those Spanish classes; gone on a date with that cute pharmacy student; campaigned for the candidate who lost by just a few votes; gone swimming with her daughter. There are places she might have gone: an Italian restaurant, the wilds of Patagonia, a Jamaican beach.

But the woman with depression stayed where she was, immobilized by an invisible force. Time passed and is now lost. Friends have disappeared. Maybe she has lost a job or a marriage.

It's natural to be awash with the question: what might have been? But the more vital question is: How can I accept my losses and move on?

Since God did not make us angels, we must put up with our human nature and be satisfied with the level of purity which, humanly speaking, we can deliver.

Saint Jane de Chantal

GOD'S EYES

The movie "Les Miserables" was playing at the local cinema and, after reading terrific reviews, my husband and I rushed out to see it. I was happy to finally be able to rush anywhere.

On the screen, the gorgeous prostitute Fantine, played by Uma Thurman, lay dying. "I'm just a whore," she mutters. Jean Valjean, played by Liam Neeson, shakes his head, "No," he says firmly, "you've never been anything but a beautiful woman in God's eyes."

My body collapsed, and I struggled to swallow the sobs that were rising from my belly. It was as if God had said the words directly to me. Damaged in ways I was not aware of, I needed desperately to hear them.

There were more tears on my pillow that night, but by then they were tears of happiness and gratitude to my loving God.

I saw full clearly that as God made us He loved us;
which love was never slacked, nor ever shall be.
And in this Love our life is everlasting.

Blessed Julian of Norwich

KEEP TRYING

Emma and I have the same spiritual mentor. Emma says that when she was a child, sixty-odd years ago, there was a great gulf between God and people. "We were His people to be sure," Emma says, her knitting needles clicking in her hands. "We learned that in school. But He seemed like such a far-away fellow." For her, she says, God was the classic bearded old gentlemen sitting on a cloud, his face marked by sternness.

By now Emma has been to enough Jesus seminars and feminist spirituality conferences to know that God loves us and lives within us. She has read the wise words of Dorothee Soelle that the distance between us and God is so blurry as to not be there.

But Emma cannot feel it. "I think I've had low-level depression all my life," she says, "and it gets in the way."

She smiles. "But I'll keep trying."

I who am Divine am truly in you.
I can never be sundered from you:
However far we be parted,
never can we be separated.
I am in you and you are in Me.
We could not be any closer.
We two are fused into one,
poured into a single mould.
Thus, unwearied, we shall remain forever.

Mechtild of Magdeburg

PURE JOY

The paint is viscous, oily, shiny. It goes thickly on the canvas, indigo and purple spreading themselves over the white. In the blue, there are tantalizing hints of hunter green, mustard, stone gray, and even a little russet.

In the strong smell of the oil there is a call to creativity and diligence — the twin sisters that make art.

The brush pushes the paint one way, then pulls it in another direction. The movements of my hand are directed by a force beyond understanding. With twists of the pallet knife, ridges and lines appear in the paint. Free form becomes shape, and things begin to emerge that I did not even know I knew.

The paint turns into a cardinal, her scarlet feathers begging to be touched. It then becomes an ash tree, its lime-colored leaves almost singing.

It draws me in until there is nothing else in the world; this is the world of creativity and creation. It is pure joy.

For me, prayer is an upward leap of the heart, an untroubled glance towards heaven, a cry of gratitude and love which I utter from the depths of sorrow as well as from the heights of joy.

Saint Thérèse of Lisieux

THE LOVE OF GOD

Many centuries ago, in a cold cell on a forlorn English coast, Julian of Norwich had a vision of God's love in which she saw its consistency and depth in a way that blew her mind. The love of God touched her heart in a way she had never felt it, and she knew that feeling would be everlasting.

God loves us women who suffer from depression, but so many of us feel we have to earn this love.

Wendy, my small ginger kitten, lay dozing on the couch one day. She stretched and yawned, then opened her sleepy eyes. She wiggled onto my legs, curled under me. Then she pushed her little face into my body, snuggling. She promptly fell back to sleep.

My heart nearly burst with love for her.

I suddenly realized Wendy did nothing to earn my love. It was hers for the taking. I loved her because she existed, and she was my cat, and that was that.

Suddenly, as I imagine it happened to Julian of Norwich, I understood completely both how and why God loves us. It wasn't only my head that knew this; my heart knew it too. I also know that you can discover this as well in your own life, and so I can end this little book, from Julian to me to you to all women who suffer depression.

*In morning, let us wake in love. All day long
let us surrender ourselves to love, by doing the will
of God, under his gaze, with him, in him, for him.
When evening comes, let us go to sleep
still in love.*

Blessed Elizabeth of the Trinity

POSTSCRIPT

It is over. What is over?
  Nay, how much is over truly:
Harvest days we toiled to sow for;
  Now the sheaves are gathered newly,
  Now the wheat is garnered duly.

It is finished. What is finished?
  Much is finished known or unknown:
Lives are finished; time diminished;
  Was the fallow field left unsown?
  Will these buds be always unblown?

It suffices. What suffices?
  All suffices reckoned rightly:
Spring shall bloom where now the ice is,
  Roses make the bramble sightly,
  And the quickening sun shine brightly,
  And the latter wind blow lightly,
And my garden teems with spices.

Christina Georgina Rossetti

EPILOGUE

Episodes of serious depression took over my life three times. These were discrete, distinct. The last was over four years ago and I have enjoyed life as never before ever since. Having emerged from these episodes, I feel that I have lived with a low-grade depression for many years, from my adolescence, onwards, if not before. The origins of my disease remain mysterious. But there are possible clues as to why depression visited me. Was it the history of mental illness on one side of the family? The preponderance of alcoholism — perhaps a form of self-medication — on the other side? Was it the result of childhood trauma or chronic stress? Or maybe my depression was caused by none of these things. It's quite possible I was simply born without sufficient psychological or physiological infrastructure to withstand many of the pressures of life. In young adulthood, I also developed a chronic medical disorder that resulted in multiple surgeries and hospitalizations. My most severe depressive episodes seemed to precede flare-ups of this condition, providing warnings that I often failed to heed. My depression may have been part and parcel of this illness; despite all my wondering, it may be that simple.

People with depression tend to ruminate on the reasons this disease chose them, and I did as well. Chinese medicine tells us that sickness is not caused by one factor alone but by a confluence of factors. This makes sense. Depression may well be the result of some combination of things: genetics; environmental factors, such as ongoing poverty; emotional issues like a parent's death; or traumatic events, such as physical abuse or a horrific car accident; and so on. I know that it is a physical illness, a very real one with known identifiable symptoms. While there are things a sufferer can to help herself both during and after bouts, she can no more cure her disease than a fish can live on land.

More recently I have turned away from the why and focused on the actual experience of depression itself: what it was like to live with and through, and what can help to heal it. I have to leave the why of it behind, since there is no definitive answer: a CT scan can't tell you why you got depression.

I took various anti-depressants, none of which had much effect (this is not to say that such medication would not help others). My depressive episodes had a tendency to lift spontaneously, possibly because they were linked to my other illness. Early on, I went to a twelve-step program for about a year, which helped, as did books like *An Adult Child's Guide to What's "Normal"* by John Friel and Linda Friel. Several rounds of counseling were useful, in an incremental manner, over a period of many years. Cognitive therapy was most helpful, leading me toward more functional analysis and away from negative thinking and low self-esteem. I would not, however, have been able to take part in cognitive therapy when depression had me at my lowest ebb. This therapy didn't cure depression, and in fact came after my last bad episode had ended. It has, however, helped prevent relapses. Meanwhile, thanks to skilful specialists, my own fortitude and possibly some luck, my other illness is in a promising remission.

I also learned how to have fun, which is something that might not come naturally to women with depression; I developed absorbing hobbies like painting, cooking, baking, and reading adventure stories set in the Antarctic and other exotic locales. My husband and I went on many fun holidays. As I am a mom now, my little daughter reminds and teaches me to play every day. Her exuberance is a refreshing, infectious tonic.

Also restorative were important adult relationships that good health has allowed me to develop. Chief among these is my relationship with my husband, Paul. Through the darkest episodes Paul never seemed to lose sight of my spirit and thus he helped me not to do so. Although depression inevitably causes tension in the home, Paul has been a continual source of love and affection. Other friends stood by, too, with patience, kindness, and understanding. One friend once challenged me, taking me to task for not keeping in touch while I was sick; I took her expectation on board, and it proved very useful, making it easier for me to put my life back together when depressive episodes passed, as they always did. I got so many good pointers from the support groups

I joined during two different episodes as well as the twelve-step group I took part in. In my work with Indigenous people in Canada, I noticed and learned from numerous examples of resilience and strength: men, youth, even toddlers, and, of course, women. The people who inspired me became valuable reference points as I struggled to get well and remain well. I encourage all women with depression to surround themselves with supportive people and especially with people who are non-judgmental and willing to learn about the illness.

Spiritual mentoring was helpful, too, in firming up my internal foundation while taking me outside myself into relationship with God and with the Mystery that surrounds us and of which we are part. As with cognitive therapy, I would not have been able to participate in spiritual mentoring in any real way while in the midst of an active period of depression. This came later. For me maintaining — or trying to maintain — a spiritual practice acts as a something of a prophylactic against depression, the words of the women mystics are potent medicine. I hope that it may be so for you as well.

It was during a spiritual mentoring session that I suddenly realized my depression is a gift. I lack the words to explain what I mean by this, only that I'm not referring to the notion of suffering as holiness. No, my depression taught me something I don't yet fully understand — something about the oneness of humanity and about the very essence of being human. It has always brought me back to myself, as nothing else can, stripping me down to the person so lovingly created by God and so loved by God.

Maura Hanrahan
St. John's, Newfoundland and Labrador, Canada
May 2009

ACKNOWLEDGMENTS

Thanks to Paul; Jemma; family and friends, especially Dolores and Regina; the many Indigenous people with whom I've worked across Canada; the counselors, therapists and other health care workers who helped me; those who write about mental illness and related issues; the twelve-step and support groups to which I belonged; the Lantern Community; and ACTA.

A special thank you to the Presentation Sisters, Newfoundland and Labrador, who supported this project with a writing grant.

WOMEN QUOTED HERE

A leading Russian poet, **Anna Akhmatova** (1889-1966) was a witness to the signs of the times. Her first husband was killed by the Bolsheviks and her son and third husband were jailed during the Stalinist era. Anna was not permitted to publish through the same period.

Welshwoman **Ann Griffiths** (1776-1805) was a Methodist mystic and poet. She left us 34 hymns that testify to the love of God.

An Italian noblewoman who was forced into an unhappy marriage, **Saint Catherine of Genoa** (1447-1510) changed her life after a mystical experience. She became devoted to the sick, in particular the victims of the plague, and was eventually joined by her husband in her work.

Saint Catherine of Siena (1347-1380) was the second youngest in a family of 25 children. She developed her religious vocation at age six and later became a Dominican nun. Although Catherine was illiterate for most of her life, she had an impact on the religious politics of her day and composed many memorable letters and prayers.

From an accomplished family with Italian roots, Englishwoman **Christina Georgina Rossetti** (1830-1894) wrote many spiritual poems and essays. She was inventive in her exploration of suffering.

A Finn of Swedish origins, the poet **Edith Södergran** (1892-1923) experienced a direct relationship with God. She died of tuberculosis at only 31.

Born in England, **Edwina Gateley** is a poet who also ministers to marginalized and abused women in Chicago. She is the founder of the Volunteer Missionary Movement.

Saint Elisabeth of Schönau (1129-1165) was a German Benedictine nun who suffered greatly with physical illness and mental anguish. Her visions of Jesus, Mary and various saints and angels were recorded on wax tablets and later in book form.

A French Carmelite who died at only 26, **Blessed Elizabeth of the Trinity** (1880-1906) is known for her idea that God dwells within. She is the author of meditations focused largely on the Trinity.

An independent thinker and artist, American poet **Emily Dickinson** (1830-1886) resisted the evangelical Christianity of her time. Many of her 1776 poems powerfully explored heaven and death.

The French Beguine lived in the late 13th century and wrote "The Soul Speaks" when she was near death.

Hadewijch, sometimes called Hadewijch of Antwerp, was a 14th-century Flemish beguine who saw God as feminine love. Very little is known about her life.

Blessed Blessed Hildegard of Bingen in Germany (1098-1179) was an extremely accomplished Benedictine abbess. She was an intellectual as well as a mystic; she was also an early ecologist, author, and political critic.

Saint Jane de Chantal (1572-1641) was the French founder of the\ Order of the Visitation of the Blessed Virgin Mary. A widow and the mother of four surviving children, Jane struggled with depression and was close to Francis de Sales.

We know little of **Blessed Julian of Norwich** (1342-1423) — not even her real name — except that she was an Englishwoman and a well-educated anchorite. The author of *Revelations of Divine Love*, she saw God as a loving mother.

A ninth century native of Constantinople, **Saint Kassiane** is the only Byzantine woman whose writing is included in the Eastern Orthodox liturgy. Kassiane was a rebel and a feminist to the core; she wrote "I hate silence when it is time to speak."

Margery Kempe (1373-1438) sought spiritual direction from Julian of Norwich and was herself the author of the first English-language autobiography. *The Book of Margery Kempe* is an account of her pilgrimages to holy sites in Europe and Asia. Married, Margery was the mother of 14 children.

Marguerite Porete, a French beguine, was burned at the stake in 1310 for heresy. Her book, *Mirror of Simple Souls*, written over ten years, is a treatise on divine love.

Maria Domitilla Galluzzi (1595-1671), an Italian nun, experienced visions of Christ's Passion. Although her spiritual life was influenced by Ignatius Loyola, she was investigated for heresy. Her writing reveals an almost sensual relationship with God.

Saint Mechtilde von Hackeborn (1240 or 41-1298) was a German Benedictine from a powerful aristocratic family. At seven, she entered the monastery, as had her older sister, the Abbess Gertrude von Hackeborn. The Helfta monastery, where the sisters lived, became a centre of German mysticism.

Born in 1207, **Mechtild of Magdeburg** was a beguine who eventually entered a convent in her native Germany. She is known for her energetic poetry, often describing God as a lover.

A Spaniard, **Saint Paula Montal** (1799-1889) was an educator and the founder of the Daughters of Mary (Pious School Sisters). Her schools are now on four continents.

Saint Teresa of Avila (1515-1582) was a Spanish Carmelite nun who suffered from poor health and wrote a powerful autobiography, *Interior Castle*.

Born Juanita Fernández Solar, **Saint Teresa of Los Andes**, was a Chilean Carmelite nun. She died of typhoid fever at only age 20 and is one of South America's dearest saints.

Saint Thérèse of Lisieux (1873-1897), known as the "Little Flower," is one of the most beloved saints. After much suffering, she died, a cloistered Carmelite, at age 24. Thérèse felt that she had a vocation to be priest, one that could never be fulfilled because of her gender.

SELECTED
BIBLIOGRAPHY

Bangley, Bernard (Ed.) (2005) *Butler's Lives of the Saints*. Brewster, MA: Paraclete Press.

Dreyer, Elizabeth A. (2005) *Passionate Spirituality: Blessed Hildegard of Bingen and Hadewijch of Brabant*. New York/Mahwah, NJ: Paulist Press.

Flinders, Carol Lee (1993) *Enduring Grace: Living Portraits of Seven Women Mystics*. New York: HarperSanFrancisco.

Gateley, Edwina (1998) *A Mystical Heart*. New York: Crossroad Publishing Co.

Gateley, Edwina (1996) *There Was No Path, So I Trod One*. Gallatin, TN: Source Books.

Hirschfield, Jane (Ed.) (1994) *Women in Praise of the Sacred: 43 Centuries of Spiritual Poetry by Women*. New York: HarperPerennial.

Madigan, Shawn, C.S.J. (Ed.) (1998) *Mystics, Visionaries, and Prophets: A Historical Anthology of Women's Spiritual Writings*. Minneapolis, MN: Fortress Press.

Porete, Marguerite (1993) *The Mirror of Simple Souls*. Mahwah, NJ: Paulist Press.

Södergran, Edith (1984) *Complete Poems*. Tr. David McDuff. Tarset, UK: Bloodaxe Books.

Spearing, A.C. (Ed.) (1998) *Julian of Norwich: Revelations of Divine Love*. Tr. Elizabeth Spearing. London: Penguin.

Spearing, Elizabeth (2002) *Medieval Writings on Female Spirituality*. New York: Penguin.

Wright, Wendy M. and Joseph F. Power, O.S.F.S. (Eds.) (1988) *Francis de Sales, Jane de Chantal: Letters of Spiritual Direction*, Tr. Péronne Marie Thibert, V.H.M. Mahwah, NJ: Paulist Press.

Wiethaus, U. (Ed.) (1993) *Maps of Flesh and Light: The Religious Experience of Medieval Women Mystics*. Syracuse, NY: Syracuse University Press, 1993.